The Delicious and Tasty Keto Vegan Recipe Collection

Super easy Keto Vegan Recipes

Nancy Graham

Please consult a licensed professional before attempting any techniques outlined in this book.

By reading this document, the reader agrees that under no circumstances is the author responsible for any losses, direct or indirect, which are incurred as a result of the use of information contained within this document, including, but not limited to, — errors, omissions, or inaccuracies.

TABLE OF CONTENTS

Low-carb coconut hamburger buns

Preparation Time: 10 minutes - Cooking Time: 20 minutes - Servings: 4

Ingredients:

- 1/2 cup coconut flour - 1 1/2 cups mozzarella cheese, shredded
- 2 tablespoons cream cheese, softened - 2 tablespoons flax meal
- 2 eggs, large - 1 tablespoon baking powder
- 1 tablespoon sesame seeds - 1/2 teaspoon salt

Directions:

1. Preheat your oven to 380°F.
2. Using a mixing bowl, whisk your flax meal, coconut flour, salt and baking soda.
3. In another bowl, put your cream cheese and mozzarella cheese. Microwave your cheese for 45 seconds to a minute. Stir it and microwave once more until it becomes melted.
4. Beat your eggs, adding into the first bowl which has the dry ingredients. Add the cheese too to the bowl. You can use your hand mixer to make the dough.

5. Separate the dough into four equal portions. Use these portions to make the buns and sprinkle sesame seeds. Press the seeds to prevent them from falling out.

6. Line the baking sheet with parchment paper and place your buns.

7. Bake for 20 minutes or until they brown on the outside.

8. Leave them to cool.

Nutrition: Calories 218 / Carbohydrates 7.2 g / Fats 13.5 g / Protein 17 g

Low-carb dinner rolls

Preparation Time: 10 minutes - Cooking Time: 10 minutes - Servings: 6

Ingredients:

- 1 cup almond flour - 1/4 cup flaxseed, ground
- 1 cup Mozzarella, shredded - 1 oz. cream cheese
- 1/2 teaspoon baking soda - 1 egg

Directions:

1. Preheat your oven to 400°F.
2. Using a microwave-safe mixing bowl, microwave cream cheese and the mozzarella for a minute. Stir them till they become smooth.
3. Add eggs in the bowl while stirring to mix well.
4. In another clean bowl, put your almond flour, baking soda and flaxseed and mix the dry ingredients.
5. Pour your egg and cheese mix into the bowl with dry ingredients. Use your hand mixer or hands to make dough by kneading.
6. Slightly wet your hands with coconut oil or olive oil and roll your dough to six balls.
7. Top them with sesame seeds and place them on the parchment paper.
8. Bake them for 10 minutes. A golden brown look will indicate that they are done.
9. Leave them to cool.

Nutrition: Calories 219 / Carbohydrates 5.6 g / Fats 18 g / Protein
10.7 g

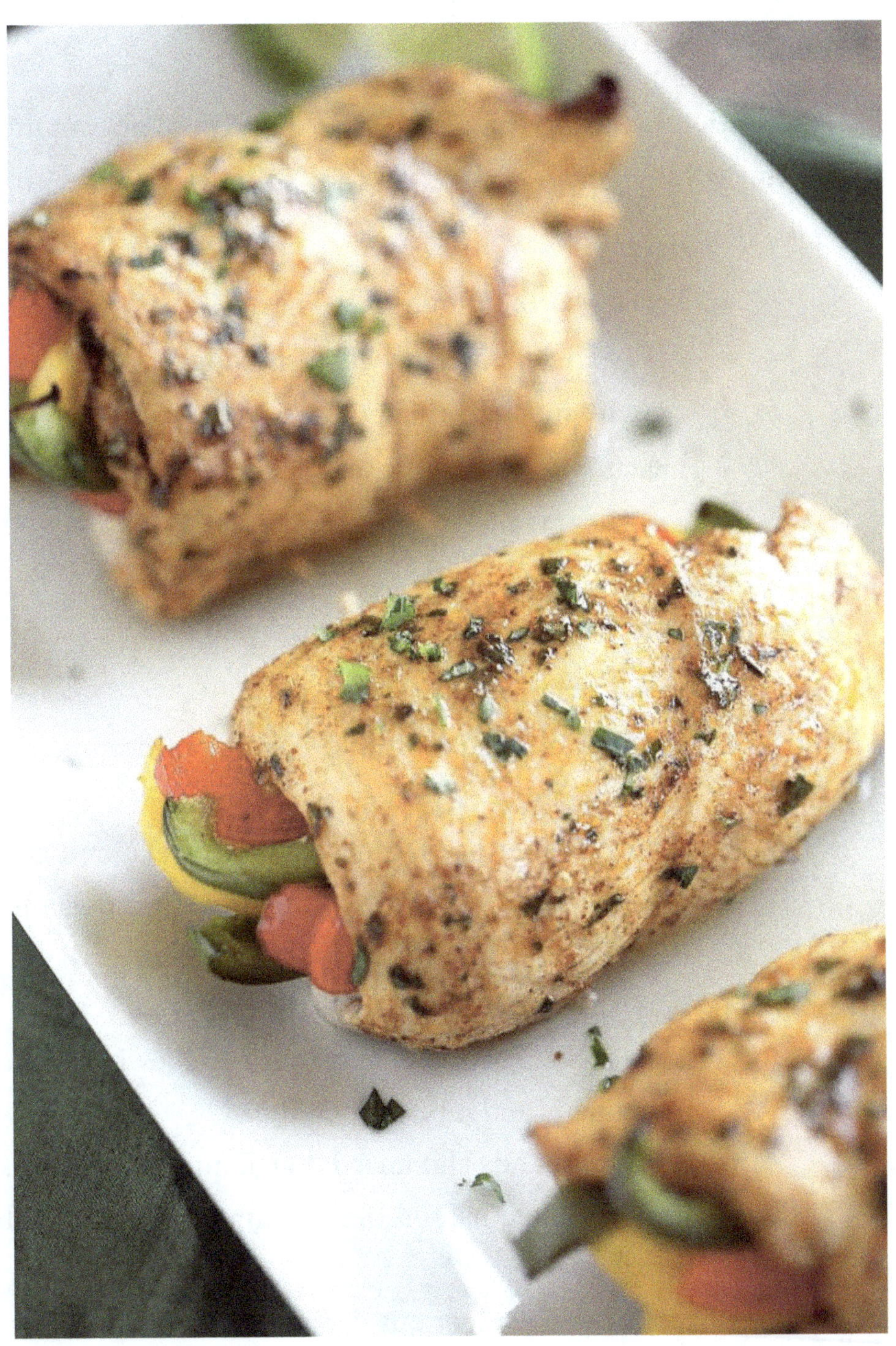

Low-carb clover rolls

Preparation Time: 10 minutes - Cooking Time: 20 minutes - Servings: 8

Ingredients:

- I/3 cup coconut flour
- 1 1/2 cup mozzarella cheese, shredded
- 1 1/2 teaspoon baking powder
- 1/4 cup parmesan cheese, grated
- 2 ounces cream cheese
- 2 eggs, large

Directions:

1. Preheat your oven to 350°F.
2. Put your almond flour and baking powder in a clean bowl and mix.
3. Using another bowl, put your Mozzarella and cream cheese and microwave for a minute. Stir it well after it melts.
4. Add eggs to the cheese and stir.
5. Add the egg-cheese mix to the bowl with dry ingredients and mix thoroughly.
6. Wet your hands and knead dough into a sticky ball.
7. Put the dough ball on the parchment paper and slice into fourths.
8. Slice each fourth or quarter into 6 smaller portions.

9. Roll each small portion into balls.

10. Roll the balls into the parmesan cheese light for them to coat it.

11. Grease your muffin pan and place 3 dough balls in each cup of the pan.

12. Bake it for 20 minutes at 350°F.

Nutrition: Calories 283 / Carbohydrates 6 g / Fats 21 g / Protein 16 g

Keto bread rolls

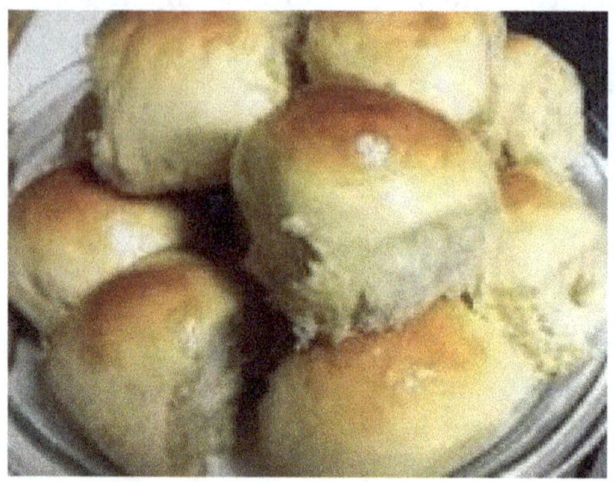

Preparation Time: 10 minutes - Cooking Time: 20 minutes - Servings: 8

Ingredients:

- 1 1/3 cups almond flour
- 1 1/2 cups shredded mozzarella cheese, part skim
- 2 oz. cream cheese, full fat
- 1 1/2 tablespoon baking powder, aluminum free
- 2 tablespoons coconut flour
- 3 eggs

Directions:

1. Preheat your oven to 350°F
2. In a clean bowl, put almond flour, coconut flour and baking powder. Mix well and set it aside.
3. Using a microwave-safe bowl, put the cream cheese and mozzarella in it and microwave for 30 seconds.

Remove the bowl, stir and microwave again for 30 seconds. This should go on until the cheese has entirely melted.

4. Using a food processor add the cheese, the eggs and flour mix. Process at high speed for uniformity of the dough. (It is normally sticky.)

5. Knead the dough into a dough ball and separate it into 8 equal pieces. Slightly wet your hands with oil for this step.

6. Roll each piece with your palms to form a ball and place each ball on the baking sheet. (should be 2 inches apart)

7. In a bowl, add the remaining egg and whisk. Brush the egg wash on the rolls.

8. Bake for 20 minutes or until they are golden brown.

Nutrition: Calories 216 / Carbohydrates 6 g / Fats 16 g / Protein 11 g

Seeded Buns

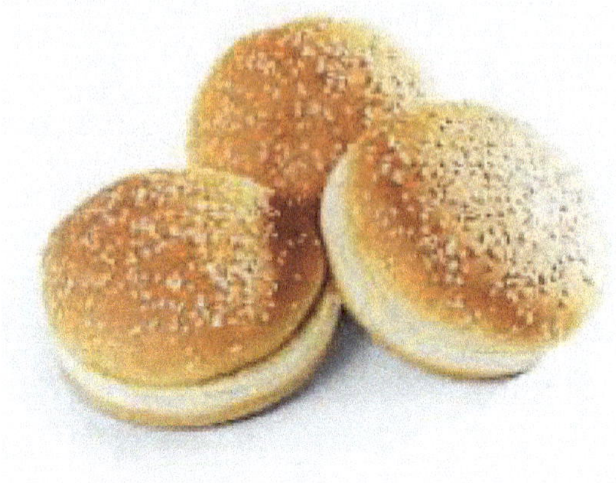

Preparation Time: 10 minutes - Cooking Time: 35 minutes - Servings: 6

Ingredients:

- 1 cup almond flour
- 2 tsp. baking powder
- 3 egg whites
- 1.25 cup hot water
- 2 tbsp. sesame seeds
- 5 tbsp. psyllium husk powder
- 1 tsp. salt
- 2 tsp. apple cider vinegar
- medium saucepan
- standard sized flat sheet

Directions:

1. Warm the water in a saucepan until it starts to bubble. Transfer to a glass dish.
2. In the meantime, prepare a flat sheet with a layer of baking lining and set to the side.
3. Blend the water with the almond flour, baking powder, psyllium husk, salt, and apple cider vinegar until it becomes a thick consistency.
4. Section into 6 equal portions and form mounds.
5. Apply pressure to flatten the mounds to approximately 1 inch thick.
6. Arrange on the prepped flat sheet and glaze with the melted butter.
7. Dust with the sesame seeds and heat for approximately 35 minutes.
8. Serve immediately and enjoy!

Nutrition: Calories 73 / Carbohydrates 7 g / Fats 3 g / Protein 3 g

Moutabelle with Keto Flatbread

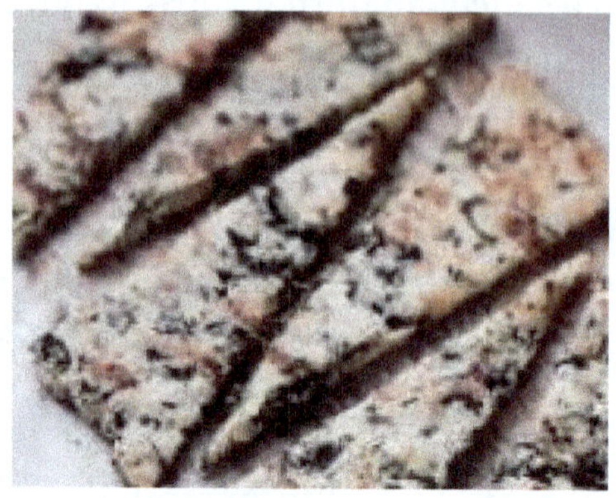

Preparation Time: 20 minutes - Cooking Time: 20 minutes - Servings: 6

Ingredients:

For the Moutabelle

- 500 grams Eggplant - 75 grams White Onion
- 10 grams Flat Parsley - 2 tbsp. tahini paste
- 2 tbsp. Lemon Juice - ¼ cup Olive Oil
- Salt, to taste - Pepper, to taste

For the Flatbread:

- ½ cup Almond Flour - 2 tbsp. Psyllium Husk
- ¼ tsp Baking Soda - pinch of Salt
- 1 tbsp. Olive Oil - 1 cup Lukewarm Water

Directions:

Prepare the Flatbread:

1. Whisk together the almond flour, psyllium husk, baking soda, and salt in a bowl.
2. Add in the water and olive oil.
3. Knead until everything comes together into a smooth dough.
4. Leave to rest for about 15 minutes.
5. Divide the dough into 6 equal-sized portions.
6. Roll each portion into a ball, then flatten with a rolling pin in between sheets of parchment paper.
7. Refrigerate until ready to use.
8. To cook, heat in a non-stick pan for 2-3 minutes per side.

Prepare the moutabelle:

9. Split each eggplant in half lengthwise. Brush with olive oil and season with salt.
10. Grill over high heat until fully cooked. Set aside until cool enough to handle.
11. Peel the grilled eggplants, and transfer the flesh to a blender or food processor. Add in remaining ingredients and process until

smooth. You may add a little warm water if it is too thick to process.

Nutrition: Calories 171 / Carbohydrates 9 g / Fats 15 g / Protein 2 g

Vegetable Latkes Spiked with Curry

Preparation Time: 15 minutes - Cooking Time: 6 minutes - Servings: 6

Ingredients:

- 100 grams Carrots, spiralized
- 100 grams Zucchini, spiralized
- 100 grams Cauliflower, minced
- 50 grams minced White Onion
- 5 grams Parsley, chopped
- ¼ cup Almond Flour
- 1 tbsp. Flax Seeds, soaked in 2 tbsp. Water
- 2 tsp Curry Powder
- ½ tsp Salt
- 2 tbsp. Olive Oil plus more for frying

Directions:

1. In a bowl, mix almond flour, egg, parsley, onions, curry powder, and salt.
2. In a non-stick skillet over medium heat, heat olive oil.
3. Using a spoon, add vegetable mixture to the hot oil, while you shape every latke like an egg ring.
4. Over medium heat, fry each side for about 3 minutes.
5. Use paper towels to drain.

Nutrition: Calories 123 / Carbohydrates 5 g / Fats 12 g / Protein 2 g

Vegan Cheese Fondue

Preparation Time: 5 minutes - Cooking Time: 20 minutes - Servings: 4

Ingredients:

- 70 grams Raw Cashews - 1 tbsp. Nutritional Yeast
- 1 tsp Garlic Powder - 2 tsp Cider Vinegar
- 2 tbsp. Gelatin - 1 tbsp. Turmeric Powder
- 1 tsp Salt - cups Water - 200 grams Zucchini, cut into sticks

Directions:

1. Boil cashews over high heat in a saucepan for 14 minutes.
2. Blend garlic powder, cashews, gelatin, vinegar, turmeric powder, water, yeast, and salt until smooth.
3. Add the puree to a saucepot and boil for about 4-5 minutes, while constantly stirring. Stir until the mixture is smooth.
4. Put it to a fondue pot and enjoy alongside zucchini sticks.

Nutrition: Calories 126 / Carbohydrates 9 g / Fats 8 g / Protein 6 g

Chocolate Peanut Butter Cookies

Preparation Time: 20 minutes - Cooking Time: 10 minutes - Servings: 14

Ingredients:

- ½ cup Peanut Butter, melted
- 3 tbsp. Coconut Oil
- ½ cup Vegan Semi-Sweet Chocolate Chips
- ½ cup Erythritol
- ½ cup Coconut Milk
- 1 tsp Vanilla Extract
- 2 cups Almond Flour
- ½ teaspoon Salt
- ½ teaspoon Baking Soda

Directions:

1. Stir together peanut butter, coconut oil, vanilla extract erythritol, and coconut milk in a bowl.
2. In a separate bowl, whisk together baking soda, flour, and salt.
3. Stir the dry mixture into the wet mixture.
4. Fold the chocolate chips in.
5. Shape dough into cookies and arrange on a baking tray lined with parchment paper.

6. Bake for 10 minutes at 375°F.

Nutrition: Calories 179 / Carbohydrates 5 g / Fats 16 g / Protein 5 g

Sweet Potato Toast

Preparation Time: 3 minutes - Cooking Time: 20 minutes - Servings: 4

Ingredients:

- 1 Ripe avocado
- 1 Large sweet potato
- Pepper and salt
- ½ cup Roughly-chopped pistachios
- 3 tbsp. Olive oil
- Crushed red pepper flakes

Directions:

1. Warm up the oven to 400°F. Prepare a baking sheet with aluminum foil.
2. Slice the potato into 1/4-inch rounds. Arrange on the baking sheet and toss it with the oil, salt, and pepper.
3. Bake for 20 minutes and garnish with the avocado and pistachios. Add a few pepper flakes.

Nutrition: Calories 132 / Carbohydrates 7 g / Fats 11 g / Protein 2 g

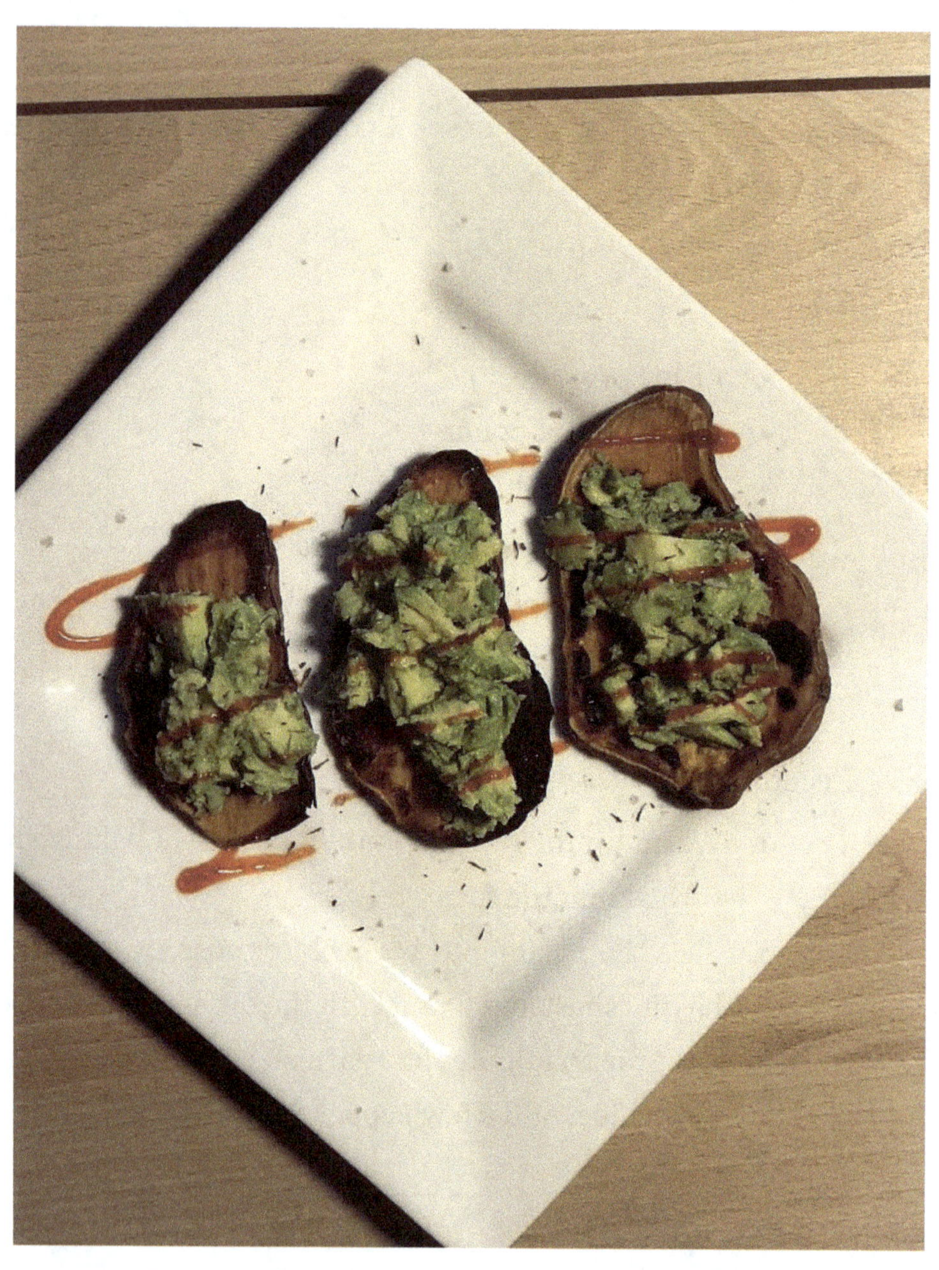

Never Fear Thin Bagels Pieces

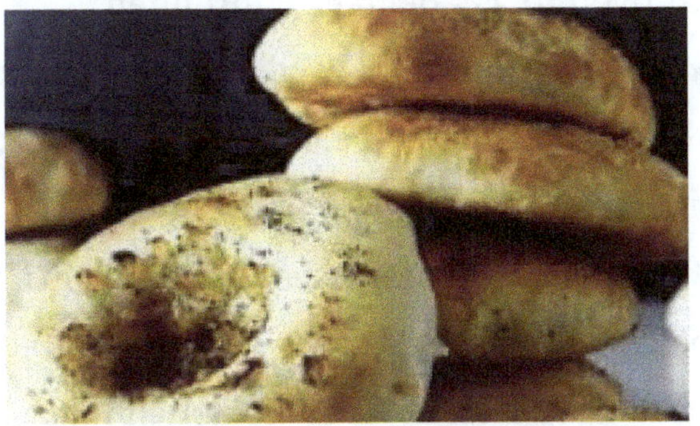

Preparation Time: 10 minutes - Cooking Time: 40 minutes - Servings: 8

Ingredients

- 3 tablespoon of ground flaxseed
- ½ a cup of tahini
- ½ a cup of Psyllium Husk powder
- 1 cup of water
- 1 teaspoon of baking powder
- Just a pinch of salt
- Sesame seeds for garnish

Directions

1. Preheat your oven to 375 degrees Fahrenheit
2. Take a mixing bowl and add Psyllium Husk, baking powder, ground flax seeds, salt and keep whisking until combined
3. Add water to the dry mix and keep mixing until the water has been absorbed fully
4. Add tahini and keep mixing until the dough forms
5. Knead well
6. Form patties from the dough that have a diameter of 4 inches and a thickness of ¼ inch
7. Lay them carefully on your baking tray
8. Cut up a small hole in the middle
9. Add sesame seeds on top
10. Bake for 40 minutes until a golden brown texture is seen
11. Cut them in half and toast if you like
12. Top them up with your favorite Keto-Vegan compliant spread
13. Enjoy!

Nutrition: Calories: 129 / Fat: 10g / Carbs: 2g / Protein: 4g

Veggie Wraps with Glorious Tahini Sauce

Preparation Time: 10 minutes - Cooking Time: 0 minutes - Servings: 8

Ingredients

- ¼ cup of sliced carrots
- 2 tablespoon of sauerkraut
- 2 tablespoon of tahini sauce

Directions

1. De-vein your leaves and wash them well
2. Add carrots, sauerkraut and wrap them up well
3. Pour the sauce directly/use as a dip
4. Enjoy!

Nutrition: Calories: 120 / Fat: 8g / Carbs: 6g / Protein: 4g

Very White Chocolate Peanut Butter Bites

Preparation Time: 110 minutes - Cooking Time: 0 minutes - Servings: 8

Ingredients

- ½ a cup of cacao butter
- ½ a cup of salted peanut butter
- 3 tablespoon of Stevia
- 4 tablespoon of powdered coconut milk
- 2 teaspoon of vanilla extract

Directions

1. Set your double boiler on low heat
2. Melt the cacao butter and peanut butter together and stir in vanilla extract
3. Take another bowl and add powdered coconut powder and Stevia
4. Stir one tablespoon at a time of the mixture into the vanilla extract mixture
5. Portion the mixture into silicone molds or lined up muffin tins and chill them for 90 minutes
6. Remove and enjoy it!

Nutrition: Calories: 77 / Fat: 7g / Carbs: 8g / Protein: 2g

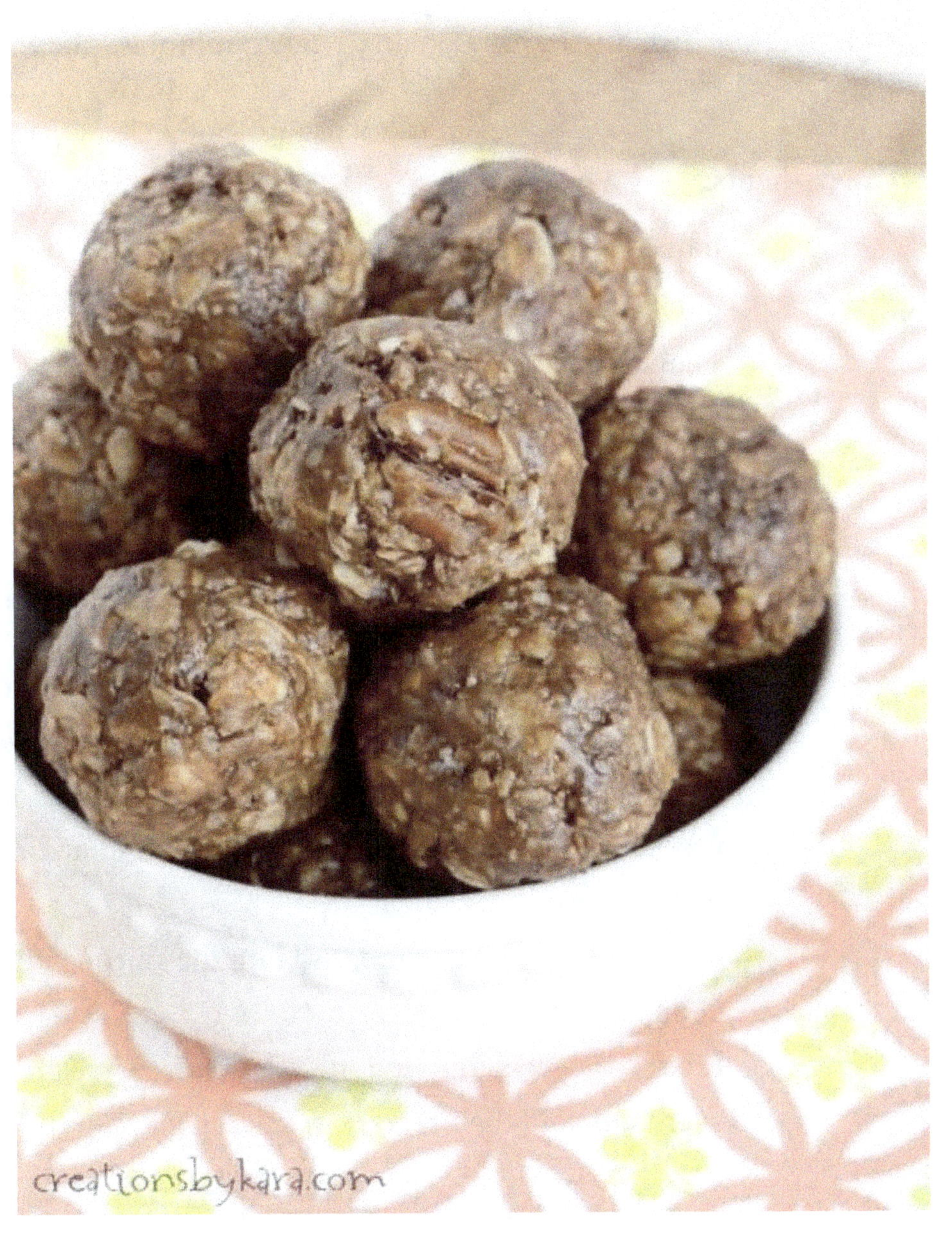

creationsbykara.com

Coconut Blueberries Ice Cream

Preparation Time: 15 min. - Cooking Time: 0 minutes - Servings: 2

Ingredients:

- half cup fresh blueberries
- 4 tbsp. shredded coconut
- 1 cup unsweetened coconut milk
- 5 tbsp. coconut butter
- 15 drops of stevia
- 2 tbsp. vanilla

Directions:

1. Pulse the blueberries, coconut milk, coconut butter, shredded coconut, stevia and vanilla using a blender.
2. Spoon the mixture into the ice cream maker and process for 1 hour or according to manufacturer's instructions.
3. Spoon the blueberries mixture into the silicone molds or an ice tray.
4. Freeze the coconut and blueberries ice cream for overnight and then serve.

Nutrition: Calories: 164 / Total fat: 29 oz. / Total carbohydrates: 9 oz. / Protein: 13 oz.

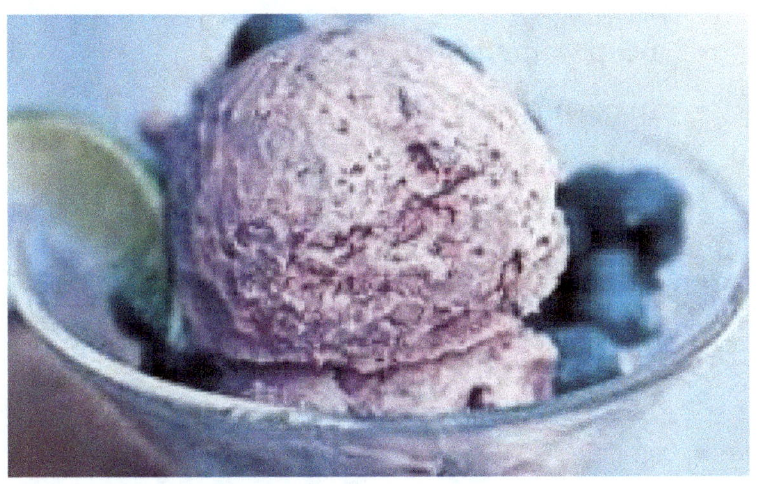

Walnuts Cakes

Preparation Time: 15 min. - Cooking Time: 5 min. - Servings: 2

Ingredients:

- 1 cup walnuts, ground
- 10 oz. unsweetened dark chocolate
- half cup coconut oil
- 7 tbsp. cocoa powder
- 3 tbsp. erythritol
- 5 tbsp. coconut butter
- 1 tbsp. vanilla
- salt

Directions:

1. Melt the coconut oil in the microwave for 5 minutes and combine it with the cocoa powder, vanilla, erythritol and salt.
2. Pour the mixture into the bowl and place in the fridge for around 10 minutes.
3. Spoon half teaspoon of coconut butter and add the walnuts and then mix well.
4. Spoon the mixture into paper muffin cups.
5. Melt the dark chocolate on medium heat for around 5 min., stirring all the time.

6. Cool the mixture and slowly pour it over the cakes.

7. The cakes should be placed in the fridge for at least 2 hours.

Nutrition: Calories: 162 / Total fat: 22 oz. / Total carbohydrates: 4 oz. / Protein: 10 oz.

Raspberries Mousse

Preparation Time: 5 min. - Cooking Time: 15 min. - Servings: 4

Ingredients:

- 1 cup fresh raspberries
- half cup almond milk
- 10 oz. coconut butter
- 3 tbsp. erythritol
- 2 tbsp. vanilla

Directions:

1. Boil the almond milk in a pan over low heat for 5 min.
2. Combine the raspberries with the almond milk and pulse well using a blender.
3. Use an electric hand mixer and beat together the raspberries mixture, coconut butter, erythritol and vanilla in a mixing bowl until the homogenous mass.
4. Pour the raspberries mixture into the jars or glasses.
5. Freeze the raspberries mixture for around 20 min. and serve.

Nutrition: Calories: 195 / Total fat: 29 oz. / Total carbohydrates: 3 oz. / Protein: 11 oz.

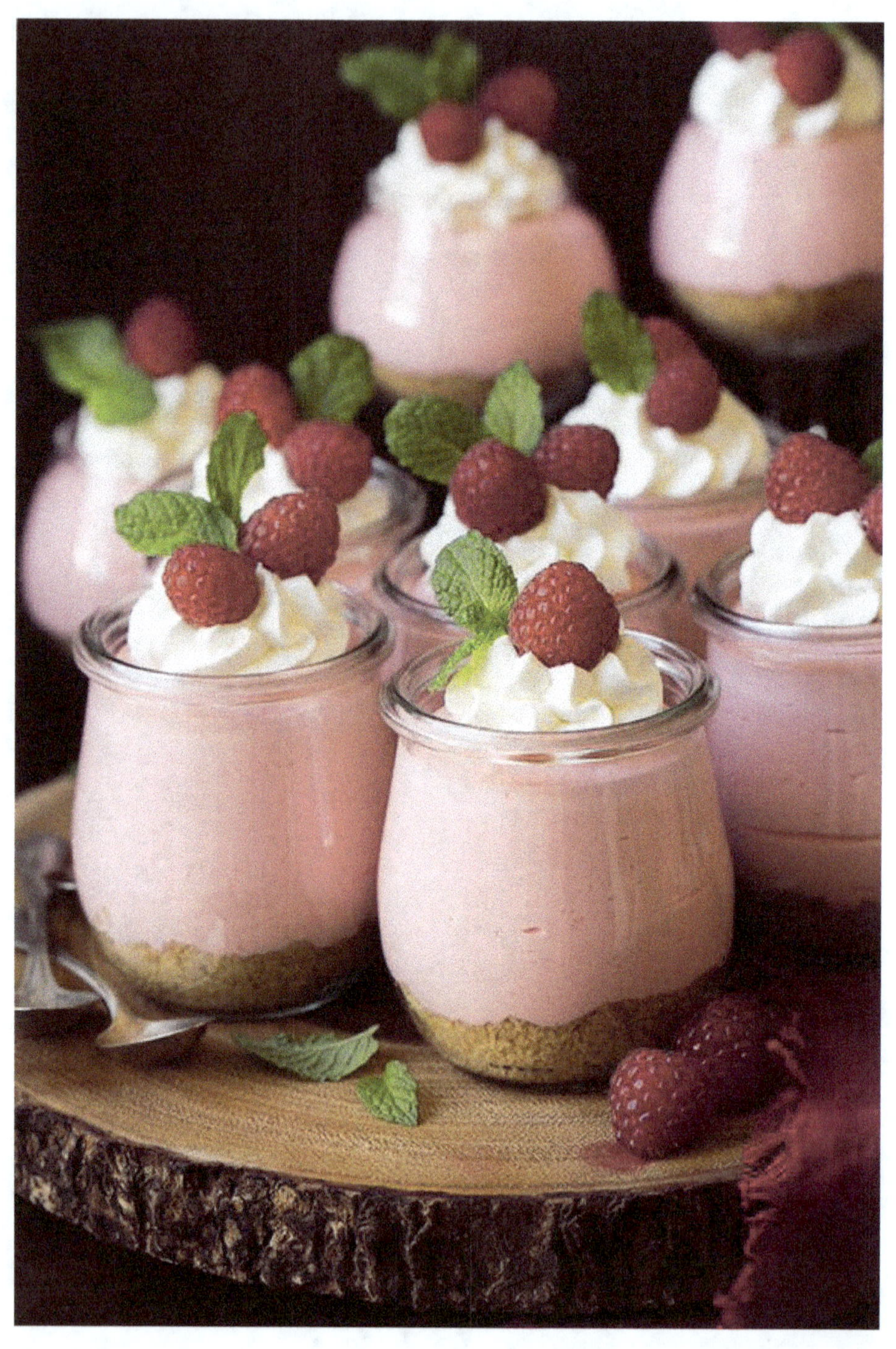

Vegan Orange Muffins

Preparation Time: 15 min. - Cooking Time: 0 minutes - Servings: 2

Ingredients:

- 2 tbsp. pure orange extract
- 2 tsp. orange zest
- 7 tbsp. coconut butter
- 5 oz. coconut oil
- 5 oz. cocoa powder
- 15 drops of stevia

Directions:

1. In a bowl, combine the coconut butter, coconut oil, orange extract, orange zest, cocoa powder and stevia.
2. Place all the ingredients into a food processor and blend until they have a smooth and creamy consistency.
3. Spoon the mixture into paper muffin cups and place in the fridge for around 2 hours and then serve.

Nutrition: Calories: 161 / Total fat: 25 oz. / Total carbohydrates: 7 oz. / Protein: 11 oz.

Coconut Keto Vegan Ice Cream

Preparation Time: 5 min. - Cooking Time: 1 h. 20 min. - Servings: 4

Ingredients:

- 15 oz. coconut cream
- 5 oz. cocoa powder
- half cup almond milk
- 4 tbsp. powdered erythritol
- shredded coconut
- vanilla

Directions:

1. Place the coconut cream, cocoa powder, shredded coconut, erythritol and vanilla into a pot and heat gently for 10 minutes, stirring, warming up until dissolved.
2. Use an electric hand mixer and whisk the almond milk and slowly pour the sweet coconut cream mixture, stirring all the time.
3. Pour the almond-coconut mixture into the pot and heat gently for 10 minutes, stirring, warming up and then cool.

4. Spoon the mixture into the ice cream maker and process for 1 hour or according to manufacturer's instructions and freeze for at least 3 hours.

Nutrition: Calories: 159 / Total fat: 29 oz. / Total carbohydrates: 6 oz. / Protein: 13 oz.

Lemon Bars

Preparation Time: 10 min. - Cooking Time: 1 h. 5 min. - Servings: 5

Ingredients:

- 4 tbsp. lemon zest, minced - 8 oz. coconut butter
- 4 tbsp. coconut cream - 1 cup almond flour
- half cup silken tofu - 4 tbsp. powdered erythritol
- 4 tsp. baking soda - vanilla

Directions:

1. Melt the coconut butter on medium heat for around 5 minutes, stirring all the time.
2. Combine the coconut butter, half cup of the almond flour, silken tofu, 2 tsp. baking soda, vanilla and 2 tbsp. of the powdered erythritol in a mixing bowl, mashing with a fork until smooth.
3. Spoon the mixture into the baking tray and bake for 30 minutes at 310 degree - 320 degree Fahrenheit.
4. Now let's start the filling by combining the lemon zest, coconut cream, remaining erythritol, baking soda and almond flour.

5. Beat together the filling mixture, in a mixing bowl, using an electric hand mixer.

6. Then, pour the lemon filling mixture onto the cooled almond crust and bake for 30 minutes at 320 degree-330 degree Fahrenheit.

7. Then cool, cut into pieces and serve with the lemon slices on top and orange juice.

Nutrition: Calories: 159 / Total fat: 49 oz. / Total carbohydrates: 9 oz. / Protein: 15 oz.

Coconut Pineapple Ice Cream

Preparation Time: 15 min. - Cooking Time: 0 minutes - Servings: 4

Ingredients:

- 3 tsp. pure pineapple extract - 1 can pineapples
- 1 cup unsweetened coconut milk - 5 tbsp. coconut butter
- 3 tbsp. erythritol - 2 tbsp. vanilla

Directions:

1. Pulse the pineapple extract, coconut milk, coconut butter, erythritol and vanilla using a blender.
2. Cut the canned pineapples into cubes and combine with the pineapple mixture.
3. Spoon the mixture into the ice cream maker and process for 1 hour or according to manufacturer's instructions.
4. Spoon the pineapples mixture into the silicone molds or an ice tray.
5. Freeze the pineapples ice cream for overnight and then serve.

Nutrition: Calories: 154 / Total fat: 34 oz. / Total carbohydrates: 8 oz. / Protein: 14 oz.

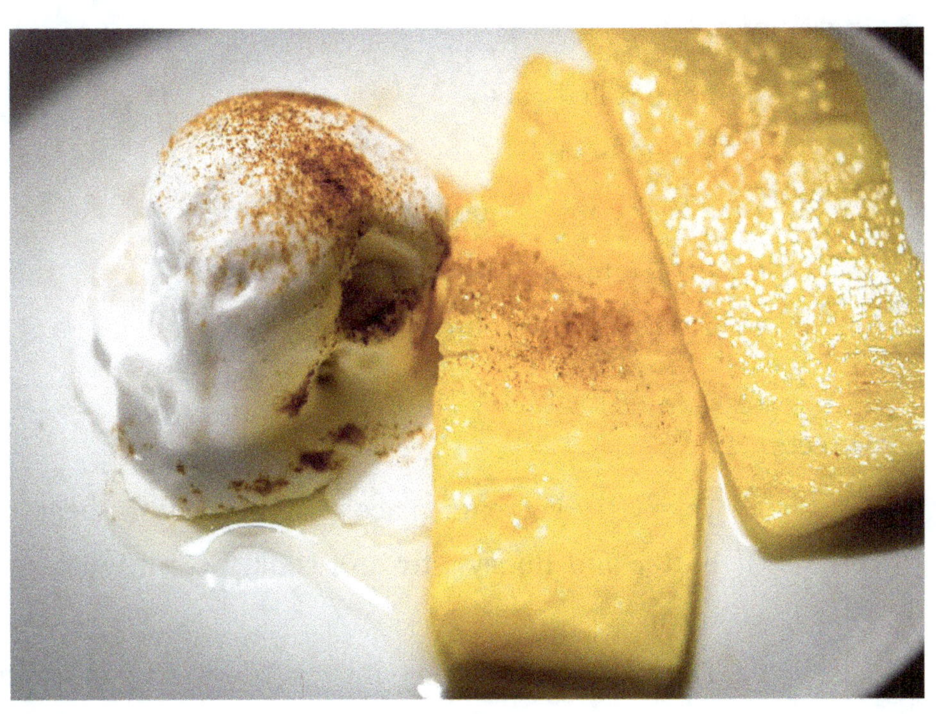

Almond Butter, Oat and Protein Energy Balls

Preparation Time: 1 hour and 10 minutes - Cooking Time: 3 minutes - Servings: 4

Ingredients:

- 1 cup rolled oats
- ½ cup honey
- 2 ½ scoops of vanilla protein powder
- 1 cup almond butter
- Chia seeds for rolling

Directions:

1. Take a skillet pan, place it over medium heat, add butter and honey, stir and cook for 2 minutes until warm.
2. Transfer the mixture into a bowl, stir in protein powder until mixed, and then stir in oatmeal until combined.
3. Shape the mixture into balls, roll them into chia seeds, then arrange them on a cookie sheet and refrigerate for 1 hour until firm.
4. Serve straight away

Nutrition: Calories: 200 Cal / Fat: 10 g / Carbs: 21 g / Protein: 7 g / Fiber: 4 g

Mango Ice Cream

Preparation Time: 5 minutes - Cooking Time: 0 minutes - Servings: 1

Ingredients:

- 2 frouncesen bananas, sliced
- 1 cup diced frouncesen mango

Directions:

1. Place all the ingredients in a food processor and pulse for 2 minutes until smooth.
2. Distribute the ice cream mixture between two bowls and then serve immediately.

Nutrition: Calories: 74 Cal / Fat: 0 g / Carbs: 17 g / Protein: 0 g / Fiber: 4 g

Chocolate and Avocado Truffles

Preparation Time: 1 hour and 10 minutes - Cooking Time: 1 minute - Servings: 18

Ingredients:

- 1 medium avocado, ripe
- 2 tablespoons cocoa powder
- 10 ounces of dark chocolate chips

Directions:

1. Scoop out the flesh from avocado, place it in a bowl, then mash with a fork until smooth, and stir in 1/2 cup chocolate chips.
2. Place remaining chocolate chips in a heatproof bowl and microwave for 1 minute until chocolate has melted, stirring halfway.
3. Add melted chocolate into avocado mixture, stir well until blended, and then refrigerate for 1 hour.
4. Then shape the mixture into balls, 1 tablespoon of mixture per ball, and roll in cocoa powder until covered.
5. Serve straight away.

Nutrition: Calories: 59 Cal / Fat: 4 g / Carbs: 7 g / Protein: 0 g / Fiber: 1 g

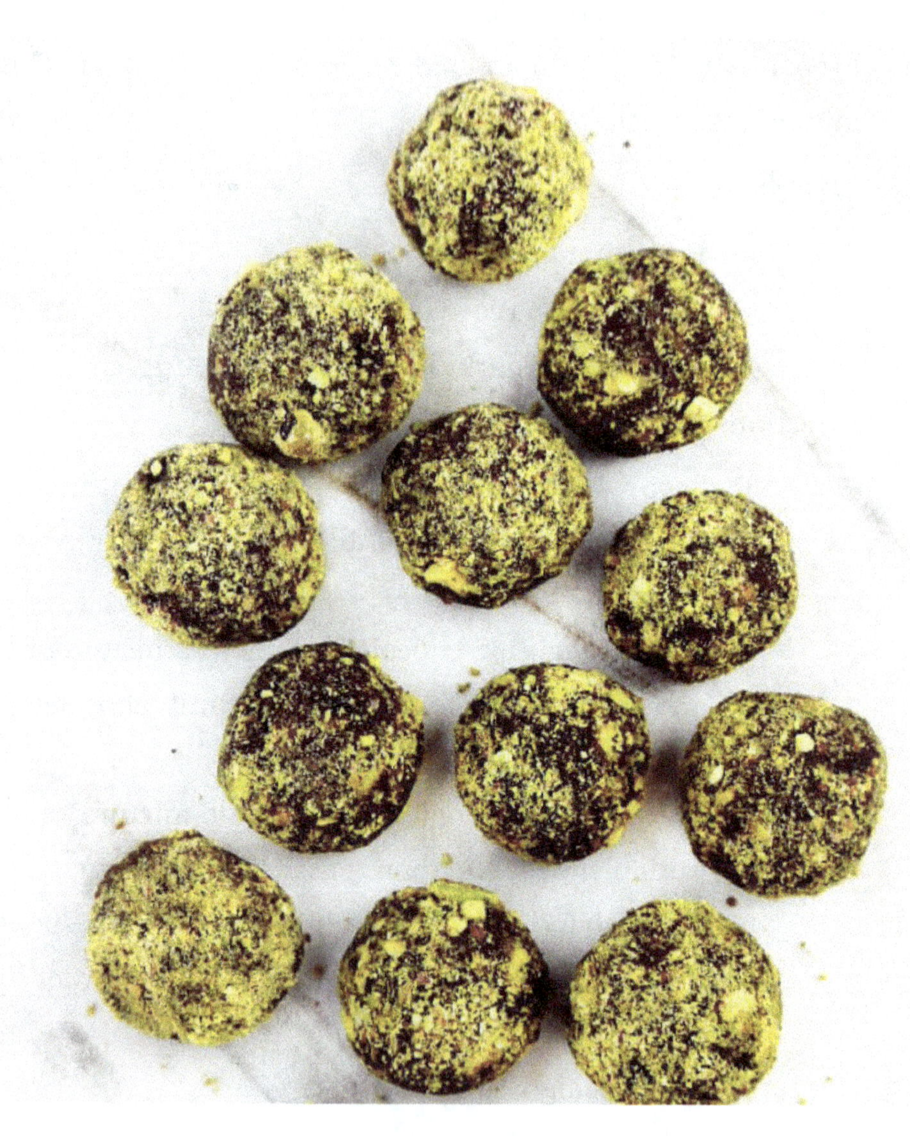

Coconut Oil Cookies

Preparation Time: 10 minutes - Cooking Time: 10 minutes - Servings: 15

Ingredients:

- 3 1/4 cup oats - 1/2 teaspoons salt
- 2 cups coconut Sugar
- 1 teaspoons vanilla extract, unsweetened
- 1/4 cup cocoa powder
- 1/2 cup liquid Coconut Oil
- 1/2 cup peanut butter
- 1/2 cup cashew milk

Directions:

1. Take a saucepan, place it over medium heat, add all the ingredients except for oats and vanilla, stir until mixed, and then bring the mixture to boil.
2. Simmer the mixture for 4 minutes, mixing frequently, then remove the pan from heat and stir in vanilla.
3. Add oats, stir until well mixed and then scoop the mixture on a plate lined with wax paper.
4. Serve straight away.

Nutrition: Calories: 112 Cal / Fat: 6.5 g / Carbs: 13 g / Protein: 1.4 g / Fiber: 0.1 g

Dark Chocolate Raspberry Ice Cream

Preparation Time: 5 minutes - Cooking Time: 0 minute - Servings: 2

Ingredients:

- 2 frouncesen bananas, sliced
- ¼ cup fresh raspberries
- 2 tablespoons cocoa powder, unsweetened
- 2 tablespoons raspberry jelly

Directions:

1. Place all the ingredients in a food processor, except for berries and pulse for 2 minutes until smooth.
2. Distribute the ice cream mixture between two bowls, stir in berries until combined, and then serve immediately.

Nutrition: Calories: 104 Cal / Fat: 0 g / Carbs: 25 g / Protein: 0 g / Fiber: 5 g

Peanut Butter and Honey Ice Cream

Preparation Time: 5 minutes - Cooking Time: 0 minute - Servings: 2

Ingredients:

- 2½ tablespoons peanut butter
- 2 bananas frouncesen, sliced
- 1½ tablespoons honey

Directions:

1. Place all the ingredients in a food processor and pulse for 2 minutes until smooth.
2. Distribute the ice cream mixture between two bowls and then serve immediately.

Nutrition: Calories: 190 Cal / Fat: 11 g / Carbs: 20 g / Protein: 4 g / Fiber: 0 g

Blueberry Ice Cream

Preparation Time: 5 minutes - Cooking Time: 0 minute - Servings: 2

Ingredients:

- 2 frouncesen bananas, sliced
- ½ cup blueberries

Directions:

1. Place all the ingredients in a food processor and pulse for 2 minutes until smooth.
2. Distribute the ice cream mixture between two bowls and then serve immediately.

Nutrition: Calories: 68 Cal / Fat: 0 g / Carbs: 17 g / Protein: 0 g / Fiber: 2 g

Almond Butter Cookies

Preparation Time: 35 minutes - Cooking Time: 5 minutes - Servings: 13

Ingredients:

- 1/4 cup sesame seeds - 1 cup rolled oats
- 3 Tablespoons sunflower seeds, roasted, unsalted
- 1/8 teaspoon sea salt
- 1 1/2 Tablespoons coconut flour
- 1/2 cup coconut sugar
- 1/2 teaspoons vanilla extract, unsweetened
- 3 Tablespoons coconut oil
- 2 Tablespoons almond milk, unsweetened
- 1/3 cup almond butter, salted

Directions:

1. Take a saucepan, place it over medium heat, pour in milk, stir in sugar and oil and bring the mixture to a low boil.

2. Boil the mixture for 1 minute, then remove the pan from heat, and stir in remaining ingredients until incorporated and well combined.

3. Drop the prepared mixture onto a baking sheet lined with wax paper, about 13 cookies, and let the cookies stand for 25 minutes until firm and set.

4. Serve straight away.

Nutrition: Calories: 158 Cal / Fat: 10 g / Carbs: 15 g / Protein: 3.4 g / Fiber: 1.8 g

Peanut Butter Fudge

Preparation Time: 50 minutes - Cooking Time: 1 minute - Servings: 8

Ingredients:

- 1/2 cup peanut butter
- 2 tablespoons maple syrup
- 1/4 teaspoon salt
- 2 tablespoons coconut oil, melted
- 1/4 teaspoon vanilla extract, unsweetened

Directions:

1. Take a heatproof bowl, place all the ingredients in it, microwave for 15 seconds, and then stir until well combined.
2. Take a freezer-proof container, line it with parchment paper, pour in fudge mixture, spread evenly and freeze for 40 minutes until set and harden.
3. When ready to eat, let fudge set for 5 minutes, then cut it into squares and serve.

Nutrition: Calories: 96 Cal / Fat: 3.6 g / Carbs: 14.6 g / Protein: 1.5 g / Fiber: 0.3 g

Coconut Cacao Bites

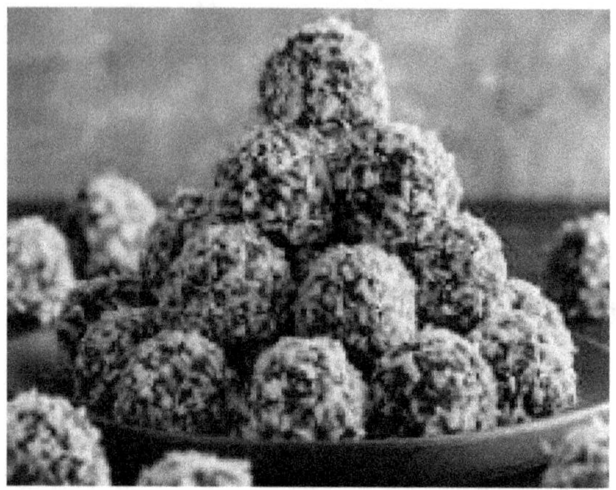

Preparation Time: 1 hour and 10 minutes - Cooking Time: 0 minute - Servings: 20

Ingredients:

- 1 1/2 cups almond flour
- 3 dates, pitted
- 1 1/2 cups shredded coconut, unsweetened
- 1/4 teaspoons ground cinnamon
- 2 Tablespoons flaxseed meal
- 1/16 teaspoon sea salt
- 2 Tablespoons vanilla protein powder
- 1/4 cup cacao powder

- 3 Tablespoons hemp seeds
- 1/3 cup tahini
- 4 Tablespoons coconut butter, melted

Directions:

1. Place all the ingredients in a food processor and pulse for 5 minutes until the thick paste comes together.
2. Drop the mixture in the form of balls on a baking sheet lined with parchment sheet, 2 tablespoons per ball and then freeze for 1 hour until firm to touch.
3. Serve straight away.

Nutrition: Calories: 120 Cal / Fat: 4.5 g / Carbs: 15 g / Protein: 4 g / Fiber: 2 g

Gingerbread Energy Bites

Preparation Time: 40 minutes - Cooking Time: 5 minutes - Servings: 14

Ingredients:

- 12 dates, pitted, chopped - 1 cup toasted pecans
- 2 ounces dark chocolate - ¼ teaspoon cloves
- 1 teaspoon ground ginger - 1 tablespoon molasses
- 1 teaspoon cinnamon - ¼ teaspoon salt
- ¼ teaspoon ground nutmeg

Directions:

1. Place all the ingredients in a food processor, except for chocolate, pulse for 2 minutes until combined.
2. Shape the mixture into 1-inch balls and place the balls on a cookie sheet lined with wax paper.
3. Place chocolate in a heatproof bowl, microwave for 2 minutes until it has melted, stirring every 30 seconds.
4. Pour the melted chocolate in a piping bag, drizzle it over prepared balls, refrigerate for 30 minutes until chocolate has hardened, and then serve.

Nutrition: Calories: 111 Cal / Fat: 2 g / Carbs: 23 g / Protein: 1 g / Fiber: 2 g

Chocolate Cookies

Preparation Time: 40 minutes - Cooking Time: 5 minutes - Servings: 4

Ingredients:

- 1/2 cup coconut oil - 1 cup agave syrup
- 1/2 cup cocoa powder - 1/2 teaspoon salt
- 2 cups peanuts, chopped - 1 cup peanut butter
- 2 cups sunflower seeds

Directions:

1. Take a small saucepan, place it over medium heat, add the first three ingredients, and cook for 3 minutes until melted.
2. Boil the mixture for 1 minute, then remove the pan from heat and stir in salt and butter until smooth.
3. Fold in nuts and seeds until combined, then drop the mixture in the form of molds onto the baking sheet lined with wax paper and refrigerate for 30 minutes.
4. Serve straight away.

Nutrition: Calories: 148 Cal / Fat: 7.4 g / Carbs: 20 g / Protein: 1.5 g / Fiber: 0.6 g

Peanut Butter Mousse

Preparation Time: 50 minutes - Cooking Time: 0 minute - Servings: 5

Ingredients:

- 3 Tablespoons agave nectar
- 14 ounces coconut milk, unsweetened, chilled
- 4 Tablespoons creamy peanut butter, salted

Directions:

1. Separate coconut milk and its solid, then add solid from coconut milk into the bowl and beat for 45 seconds until fluffy.
2. Then beat in remaining ingredients until smooth, refrigerate for 45 minutes and serve.

Nutrition: Calories: 270 Cal / Fat: 20 g / Carbs: 19 g / Protein: 5 g / Fiber: 1 g

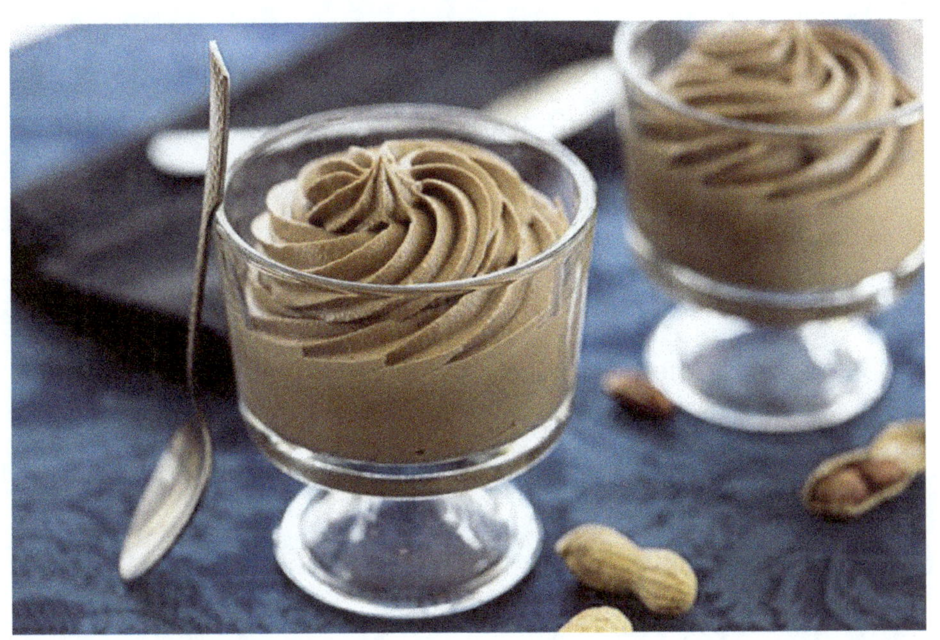

Baked Zucchini Chips

Preparation Time: 20 minutes - Cooking Time: 2 hours 45 minutes - Servings: 10

Ingredients:

- 2 medium zucchini, sliced with a mandolin
- 1 tbsp. olive oil
- 1/2 tsp salt

Directions:

1. Preheat your oven to 200 degrees F.
2. Prepare your baking sheets by lining with parchment paper.
3. Add all ingredients to a large mixing bowl and toss to coat the zucchini with oil and salt thoroughly.
4. Arrange the zucchini slices in a single layer on the baking sheet. They can touch but they should not overlap.
5. Bake for 2 and a half hours or until the zucchini chips are golden and crispy.
6. Turn off the oven and allow them to cool with the oven door cropped slightly open. This will allow the zucchini chips to crisp up even more as they cool.

Nutrition: Total fat: 1.5g / Cholesterol: 0mg / Sodium: 120mg / Total carbohydrates: 1.3g

Dietary fiber: 0.4g / Protein: 0.5g / Calcium: 6mg / Potassium: 103mg / Iron: 0mg

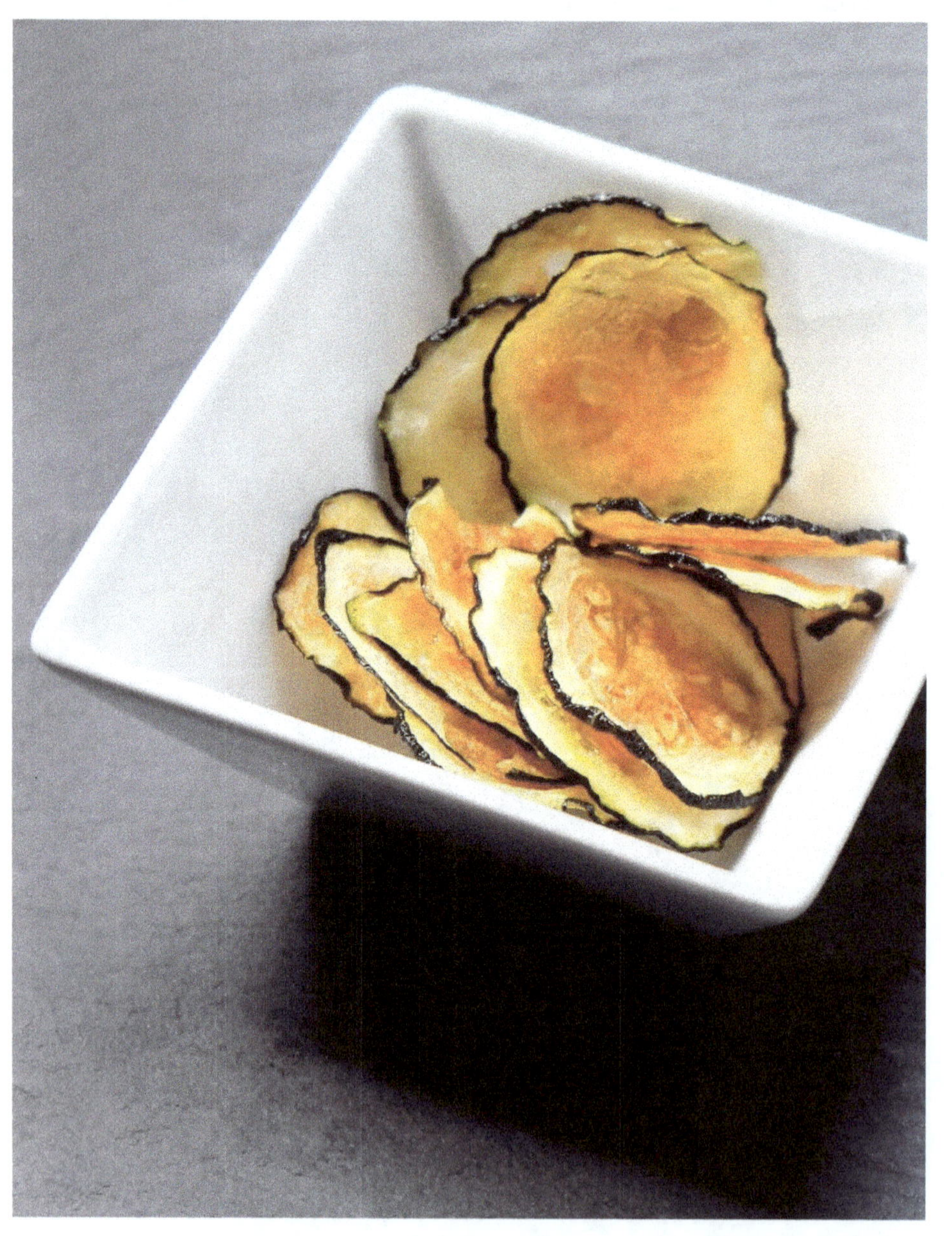

Gluten-Free Nut-Free Red Velvet Cupcakes

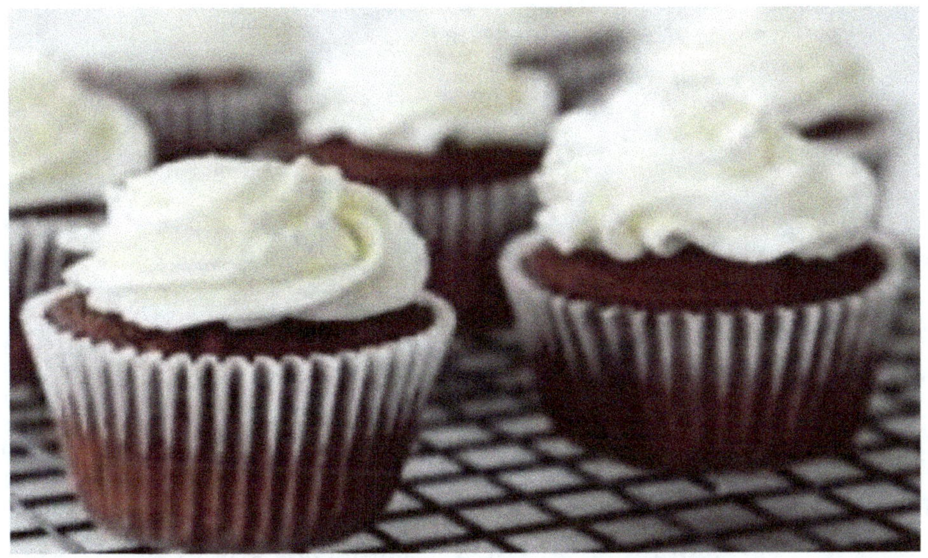

Preparation Time: 20 minutes - Cooking Time: 50 minutes - Servings: 8

Ingredients:

- 2 tbsp. flax meal
- 4 tbsp. cocoa powder
- ½ cup of almond butter
- ½ cup unsweetened almond milk
- 1 tbsp. granulated erythritol
- 2 tbsp. apple cider vinegar
- 4 tbsp. ground flaxseed

- 1 tsp baking powder
- 1/2 tsp baking soda

Directions:

1. Preheat your oven to 350 degrees F.
2. Prepare a standard size muffin tin by lining it with paper liners.
3. In a small bowl, whisk together almond butter, almond milk and apple cider vinegar until a smooth combined mixture is achieved. Stir in flax seeds and erythritol and set aside.
4. In a large mixing bowl, sift together cocoa powder, flax meal, baking powder and baking soda. Mix to combine.
5. Pour the wet mixture into the dry ingredients and stir until there are no lumps. Do not overmix.
6. Divide the batter between the lined muffin wells. Ensure that each muffin is filled 3/4 of the way. Bake for 30 minutes or until the top of each muffin is firm to the touch.
7. Remove from the oven and allow to cool in pan for 10 minutes. Remove the cupcakes from the pan and allow to cool completely. Serve.

Nutrition: Total fat: 2.9g / Cholesterol: 0mg / Sodium: 93mg / Total carbohydrates: 4.9g

Dietary fiber: 2.4g / Protein: 1.8g / Calcium: 53mg / Potassium: 196mg / Iron: 2mg

5-Ingredient Ice-cream

Preparation Time: 20 minutes - Cooking Time: 1 hour 10 minutes - Servings: 6

Ingredients:

- 1 ½ cup full fat coconut milk
- 1/3 cup natural peanut butter
- 2 tbsp. vanilla extract
- 1/8 tsp stevia powder
- A pinch of salt

Directions:

1. Prior to starting this recipe, place a freezer-safe container in the freezer for at least 24 hours before to ensure that when the ice cream mixture is transferred no ice crystals are formed.
2. Add all ingredients to a blender and blend until a smooth and creamy consistency is achieved.
3. Chill this mixture by placing it in the refrigerator for 1 hour.
4. Transfer the mixture to an ice-cream maker and churn for 10 minutes or until it achieves a soft serve consistency.

5. Transfer the ice cream to the prepared freezer-safe container and freeze for at least one hour before serving. Can be served with caramel sauce

Nutrition: Total fat: 10.1g / Cholesterol: 0mg / Sodium: 34mg / Total carbohydrates: 3.7

Dietary fiber: 0.9g / Protein: 4.7g / Calcium: 1mg / Potassium: 6mg / Iron: 2mg

Tantalizing Apple Pie Bites

Preparation Time: 20 minutes - Cooking Time: 0 minutes - Servings: 4

Ingredients

- 1 cup chopped walnuts - ½ a cup of coconut oil
- ¼ cup of ground flaxseed - ½ ounce of frozen, dried apples
- 1 teaspoon of vanilla extract
- 1 teaspoon of cinnamon - Liquid Stevia

Directions

1. Melt the coconut oil until it is liquid
2. Take your blender and add walnuts, coconut oil, and process well
3. Add flaxseeds, vanilla, and Stevia
4. Keep processing until a fine mixture form
5. Stop and add crumbled dried apples
6. Process until your desired texture appears
7. Portion the mixture amongst muffin molds and allow them to chill

Nutrition: Calories: 194 / Fat: 19g / Carbs: 2g / Protein: 2.3g

Vegan Compliant Protein Balls

Preparation Time: 20 minutes - Cooking Time: 0 minutes - Servings: 8

Ingredients

- 1 cup of creamed coconut
- 2 scoops of Vega Sport Chocolate Protein (or any protein powder of your preference)
- ¼ cup of ground flax seed - ½ a teaspoon of vanilla extract
- ½ a teaspoon of mint extract - 1-2 tablespoon of cocoa powder

Directions

1. Take a large-sized bowl and melt the creamed coconut
2. Add the vanilla extract and stir well
3. Stir in flaxseed, protein powder and knead until the fine dough forms
4. Form 24 balls and allow the balls to chill for 10-15 minutes
5. Roll them up in some cocoa powder if you prefer and serve!

Nutrition: Calories: 260 / Fat: 20g / Carbs: 3g / Protein: 10g

The Keto Lovers "Magical" Grain-Free Granola

Preparation Time: 10 minutes - Cooking Time: 75 minutes - Servings: 10

Ingredients

- ½ a cup of raw sunflower seeds
- ½ a cup of natural hemp hearts
- ½ a cup of flaxseeds - ¼ cup of chia seeds
- 2 tablespoon of Psyllium Husk powder
- 1 tablespoon of cinnamon
- Stevia - ½ a teaspoon of baking powder
- ½ a teaspoon of salt - 1 cup of water

Directions

1. Preheat your oven to 300 degrees Fahrenheit
2. Line up a baking sheet with parchment paper
3. Take your food processor and grind all the seeds
4. Add the dry ingredients and mix well
5. Stir in water until fully incorporated
6. Allow the mixture to sit for a while until it thickens up
7. Spread the mixture evenly on top of your baking sheet (giving a thickness of about ¼ inch)

8. Bake for 45 minutes

9. Break apart the granola and keep baking for another 30 minutes until the pieces are crunchy

10. Remove and allow them to cool

Nutrition: Calories: 292 / Fat: 25g / Carbs: 12g / Protein: 8g

Pumpkin Butter Nut Cup

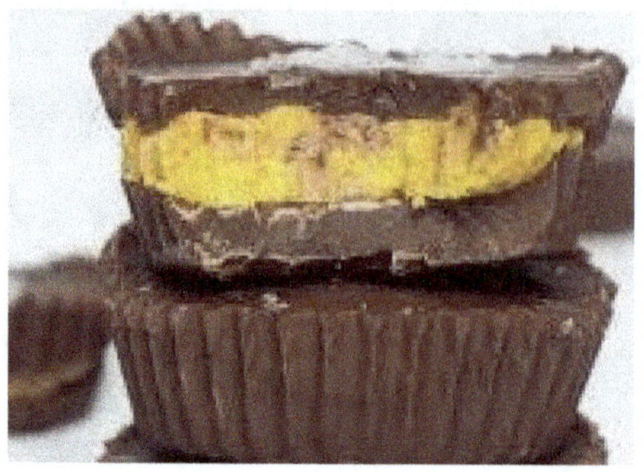

Preparation Time: 135 minutes - Cooking Time: 0 minute - Servings: 5

Ingredients:

For Filing

- ½ a cup of organic pumpkin puree
- 1/2a cup of almond butter
- 4 tablespoon of organic coconut oil
- ¼ teaspoon of organic ground nutmeg
- ¼ teaspoon of organic ground ginger
- 1 teaspoon of organic ground cinnamon
- 1/8 teaspoon of organic ground clove
- 2 teaspoon of natural vanilla extract

For Topping

- 1 cup of organic raw cacao powder
- 1 cup of organic coconut oil

Directions

1. Take a medium-sized bowl and add all of the listed ingredients under pumpkin filling
2. Mix well until you have a creamy mixture
3. Take another bowl and add the topping mixture and mix well
4. Take a muffin cup and fill it up with 1/3 of the chocolate topping mix
5. Chill for 15 minutes
6. Add 1/3 of the pumpkin mix and layer out on top
7. Chill for 2 hours
8. Repeat until all the mixture has been used up

Nutrition:Calories: 105 / Fat: 10.1g / Carbs: 3.3g / Protein: 2.9g

Unique Gingerbread Muffins

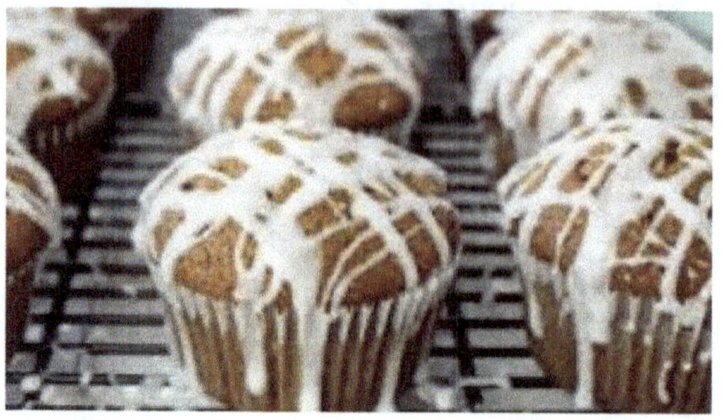

Preparation Time: 15 minutes - Cooking Time: 30 minutes - Servings: 12

Ingredients

- 1 tablespoon of ground flaxseed
- 6 tablespoon of coconut milk
- 1 tablespoon of apple cider vinegar
- ½ a cup of peanut butter
- 2 tablespoon of the gingerbread spice blend
- 1 teaspoon of baking powder
- 1 teaspoon of vanilla extract
- 2-3 tablespoon of Swerve

Directions

1. Pre-heat your oven to a temperature of 350 degrees Fahrenheit

2. Take a bowl and add flaxseeds, sweetener, salt, vanilla, spices, and coconut milk

3. Keep it on the side for a while

4. Add peanut butter, baking powder and keep mixing until combined well

5. Stir in peanut butter and baking powder

6. Mix well

7. Spoon the mixture into muffin liners

8. Bake for 30 minutes

9. Allow them to cool and enjoy!

Nutrition: Calories: 158 / Fat: 13g / Carbs: 3g / Protein: 6g

The Vegan Pumpkin Spicy Fat Bombs

Preparation Time: 100 minutes - Cooking Time: 0 minutes - Servings: 12

Ingredients

- ¾ cup of pumpkin puree
- ¼ cup of hemp seeds
- ½ a cup of coconut oil
- 2 teaspoon of pumpkin pie spice
- 1 teaspoon of vanilla extract
- Liquid Stevia

Directions

1. Take a blender and add all of the ingredients
2. Blend them well and portion the mixture out into silicon molds
3. Allow them to chill and enjoy!

Nutrition: Calories: 103 / Fat: 10g / Carbs: 2g / Protein: 1g

The Low Carb "Matcha" Bombs

Preparation Time: 100 minutes - Cooking Time: 0 minutes - Servings: 12

Ingredients

- ¾ cup of hemp sees
- ½ a cup of coconut oil
- 2 tablespoon of coconut butter
- 1 teaspoon of matcha powder
- 2 tablespoon of vanilla extract
- ½ a teaspoon of mint extract
- Liquid Stevia

Directions

1. Take your blender and add hemp seeds, matcha, coconut oil, mint extract and Stevia
2. Blend well and divide the mixture into silicone molds
3. Melt the coconut butter and drizzle them on top of your cups
4. Allow the cups to chill and serve!

Nutrition: Calories: 200 / Fat: 20g / Carbs: 3g / Protein: 5g

The No-Bake Keto Cheese Cake

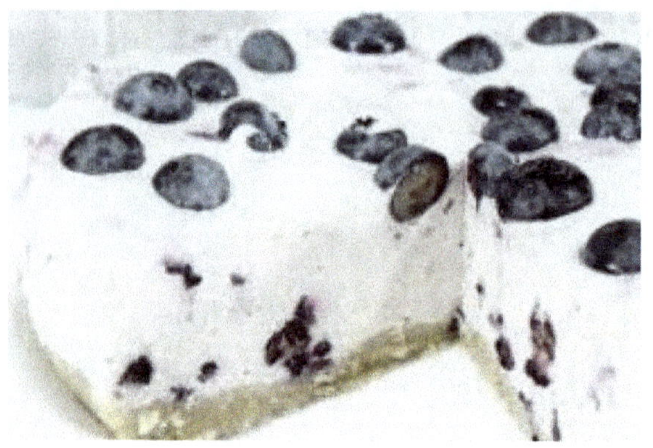

Preparation Time: 120 minutes - Cooking Time: 0 minutes - Servings: 4

Ingredients

For Crust

- 2 tablespoon of ground flaxseed
- 2 tablespoon of desiccated coconut
- 1 teaspoon of cinnamon

For Filling

- 4 ounce of vegan cream cheese
- 1 cup of soaked cashews
- ½ a cup of frozen blueberries

- 2 tablespoon of coconut oil
- 1 tablespoon of lemon juice
- 1 teaspoon of vanilla extract
- Liquid Stevia

Directions

1. Take a container and mix all of the crust ingredients
2. Mix them well and flatten them at the bottom to prepare the crust
3. Take a blender and mix all of the filling ingredients and blend until smooth
4. Distribute the filling on top of your coat and chill it in your freezer for about 2 hours
5. Enjoy!

Nutrition: Calories: 182 / Fat: 16g / Carbs: 6g / Protein: 3g

Raspberry Chocolate Cups

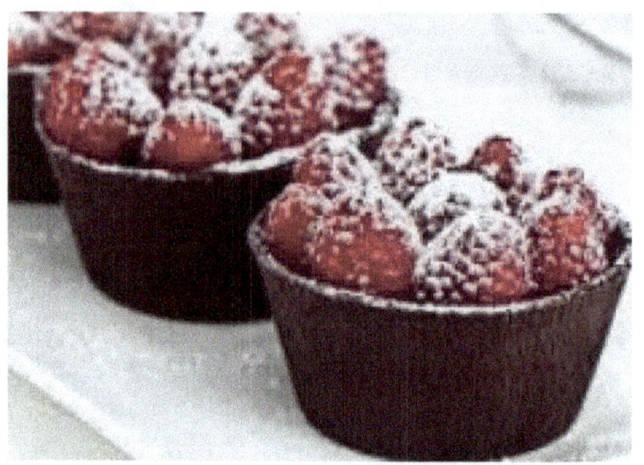

Preparation Time: 60 minutes - Cooking Time: 0 minutes - Servings: 12

Ingredients

- ½ a cup of cacao butter
- ½ a cup of coconut manna
- 4 tablespoon of powdered coconut milk
- 3 tablespoon of granulated sugar substitute
- 1 teaspoon of vanilla extract
- ¼ cup of dried and crushed frozen raspberries

Directions

1. Melt cacao butter and add coconut manna
2. Stir in vanilla extract
3. Take another dish and add coconut powder and sugar substitute

4. Stir the coconut mix into the cacao butter, 1 tablespoon at a time, making sure to keep mixing after each addition

5. Add the crushed dried raspberries

6. Mix well and portion it out into muffin tins

7. Chill for 60 minutes and enjoy it!

Nutrition: Calories: 158 / Fat: 15g / Carbs: 1g / Protein: 3g

Exuberant Pumpkin Fudge

Preparation Time: 120 minutes - Cooking Time: 0 minutes - Servings: 25

Ingredients

- 1 and a ¾ cup of coconut butter
- 1 cup of pumpkin puree
- 1 teaspoon of ground cinnamon
- ¼ teaspoon of ground nutmeg
- 1 tablespoon of coconut oil

Directions

1. Take an 8x8 inch square baking pan and line it with aluminum foil to start with
2. Take a spoon of the coconut butter and add into a heated pan; let the butter melt over low heat
3. Toss in the spices and pumpkin and keep stirring it until a grainy texture has formed
4. Pour in the coconut oil and keep stirring it vigorously in order to make sure that everything is combined nicely
5. Scoop up the mixture into the previously prepared baking pan and distribute evenly

6. Place a piece of wax paper over the top of the mixture and press on the upper side to make evenly straighten up the topside

7. Remove the wax paper and throw it away

8. Place the mixture in your fridge and let it cool for about 1-2 hours

9. Take it out and cut it into slices, then eat

Nutrition: Calories: 120 / Protein: 1.2g / Carbs: 4.2g / Fats: 10.7g

Wonderful Peanut Butter Mousse

Preparation Time: 2 to 5 minutes - Cooking Time: 0 minutes - Servings: 4

Ingredients:

- 4 tablespoons natural unsweetened peanut butter
- ½ can coconut cream
- 1 ½ teaspoons stevia

Directions:

1. First of all, please check that you've all the ingredients obtainable. Now combine all ingredients & whip for one minute, until mixture forms peaks.
2. Finally, chill for at least three hours or until a mousse texture is achieved.

Nutrition: Calories: 206 / Protein: 5 g / Fat: 18 g / Carbs: 6 g

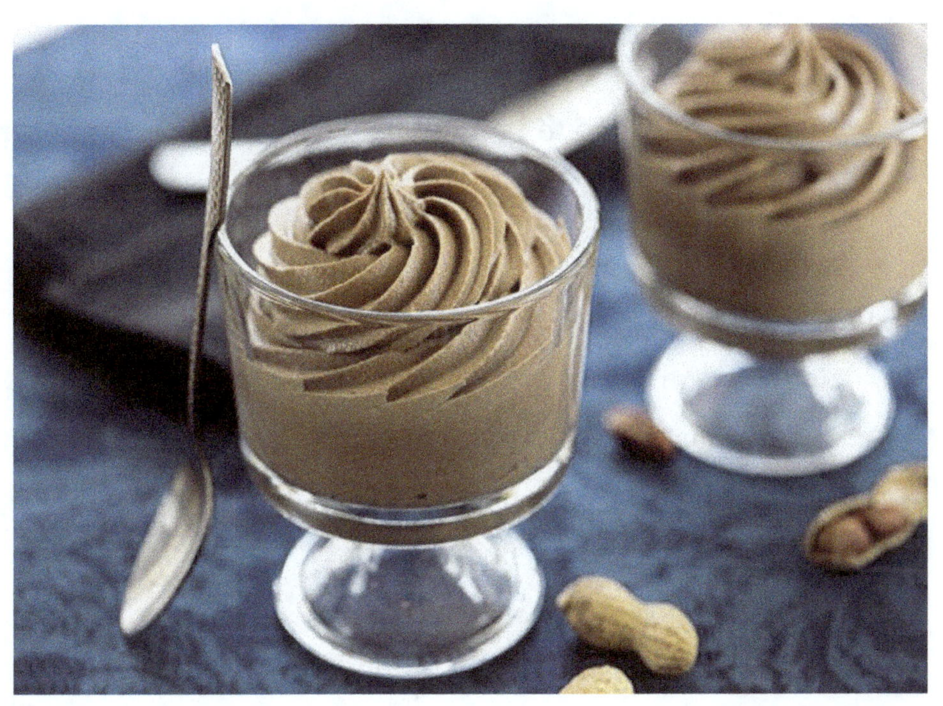

Lucky Mediterranean Style Pasta

Preparation Time: 10 to 15 minutes - Cooking Time: 5 minutes - Servings: 4

Ingredients:

- 1 cup Spinach
- Salt and black pepper to taste
- 2 ½ tablespoons Olive oil
- 2 tablespoons Butter
- 5 cloves Garlic (minced)
- ¼ cup Feta cheese (crumbled)
- ¼ cup Sun-dried tomatoes
- 2 tablespoons capers
- ¼ cup Parmesan cheese(shredded)
- 2 tablespoons Italian flat-leaf parsley(chopped)
- 10 Kalamata olives(halved)
- 2 Zucchini(spiralized)

Directions:

1. First of all, please confirm you've all the ingredients on the market. Now please heat oil and butter in a large pan& sauté the garlic, spinach, zucchini, in its seasoned with salt & pepper until the spinach wilts & zucchini becomes tender

2. Now drain any extra liquid.

3. One thing remains to be done. Now quickly add the rest of the ingredients except the cheese and stir cook properly for about 2 to 5 minutes.

4. Finally, remove from the flame & toss in the cheese.

Nutrition: Calories: 231 / Protein: 6.5 g / Fat: 20 g / Carbs: 6.5 g

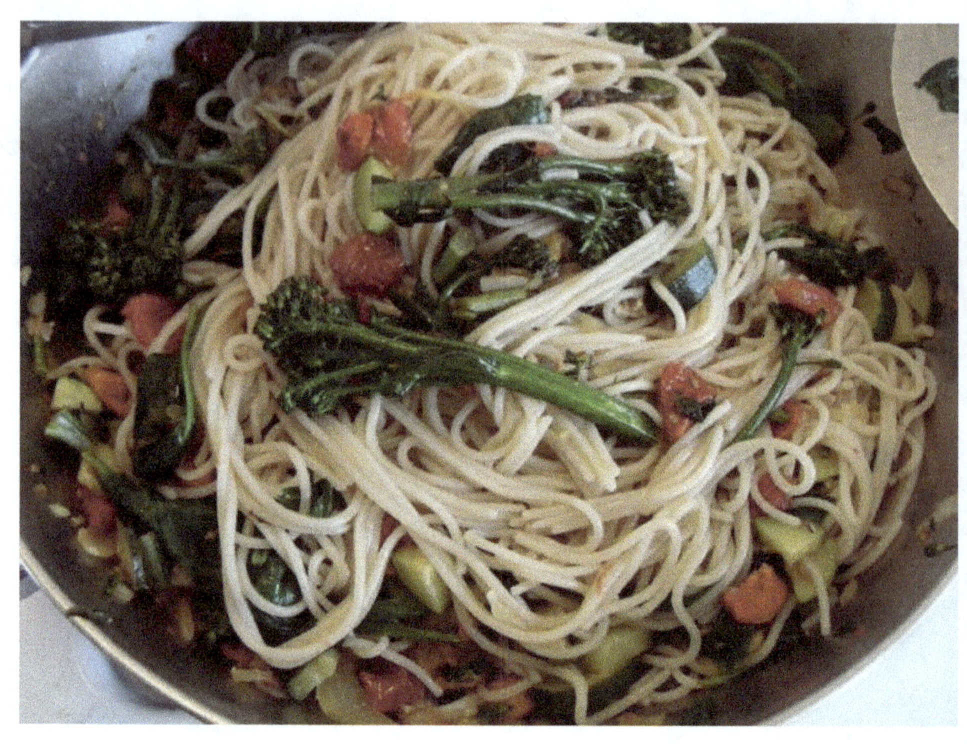

Awesome Roasted Acorn Squash

Preparation Time: 40 to 45 minutes - Cooking Time: 0 minutes - Servings: 4

Ingredients:

- ¼ teaspoon black pepper
- ¼ cup parmesan cheese, grated
- 8 fresh thyme sprigs
- 2 ½ tablespoons olive oil
- 1 large acorn squash, cut in half lengthwise

Directions:

1. First of all, please certify you've all the ingredients on the market. Preheat the oven to 4000 F. /2000 C.
2. Now remove the seed from squash & cut into ¾ slices.
3. Add squash slices, parmesan cheese, olive oil, thyme, pepper, and salt in a bowl and toss to coat.
4. One thing remains to be done. Then spread squash onto a baking tray & roast in preheated oven for about 25 to 30 minutes or until golden brown.
5. Finally, serve & enjoy.

Nutrition: Calories: 253 / Protein: 12.9 g / Fat: 16.1 g / Carbs: 11.3 g

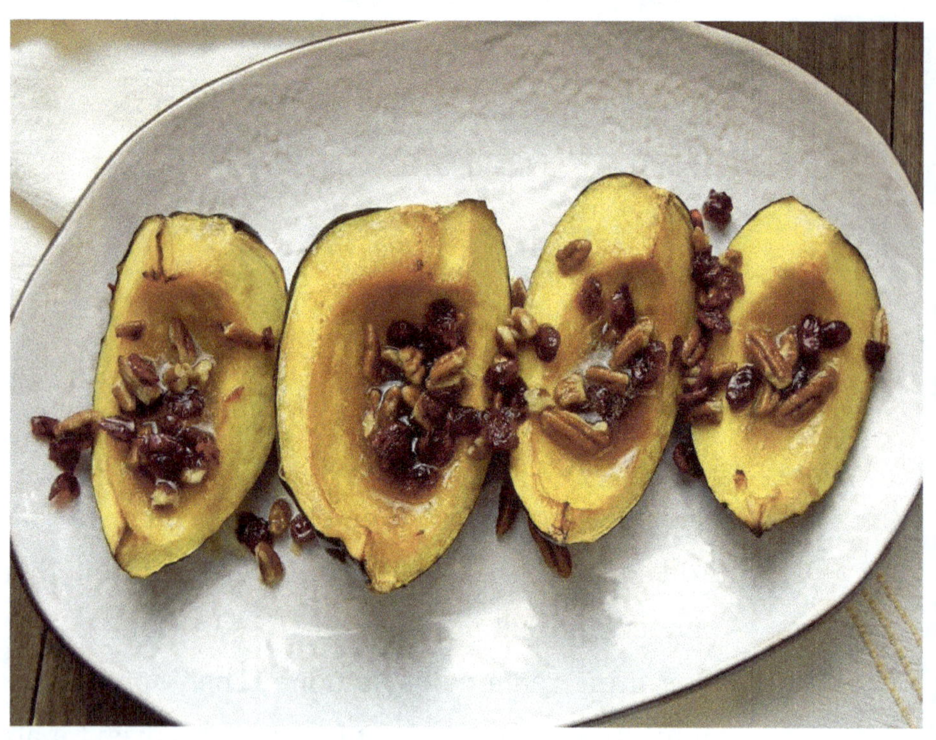

Unique Scrambled Tofu

Preparation Time: 5 to 10 minutes - Cooking Time: 0 minutes - Servings: 1

Ingredients:

- Pepper to taste - 1 ½ tablespoon grapeseed oil
- 1 tablespoon vegetable broth - ¼ teaspoon garlic powder
- 1 teaspoon nutritional yeast - 14 ounces soft tofu
- ¾ teaspoon salt - 1 teaspoon onion powder
- ¼ teaspoon turmeric powder

Directions:

1. First off all go ahead and assemble all the ingredients at one place. In a small bowl, thoroughly combine nutritional yeast, spices, salt, and pepper. Set aside.
2. Now crumble the tofu depending on how "chunky" you want the scramble to be. Set aside.
3. Please heat oil in a pan on moderate.
4. Now we can plow ahead to succeeding the most significant step. Add tofu & stir until heated through.
5. Add vegetable broth and the spice mix.
6. Now stir until the tofu is evenly coated with the spices.
7. Only one thing remains to be done now. Take off the warmth once most of the liquid is absorbed.

8. Finally, serve hot or warm. Finally, we've completed the recipe. Enjoy.

Nutrition: Calories: 256.5 / Protein: 27g / Fat: 16.2g / Carbs: 5.3g

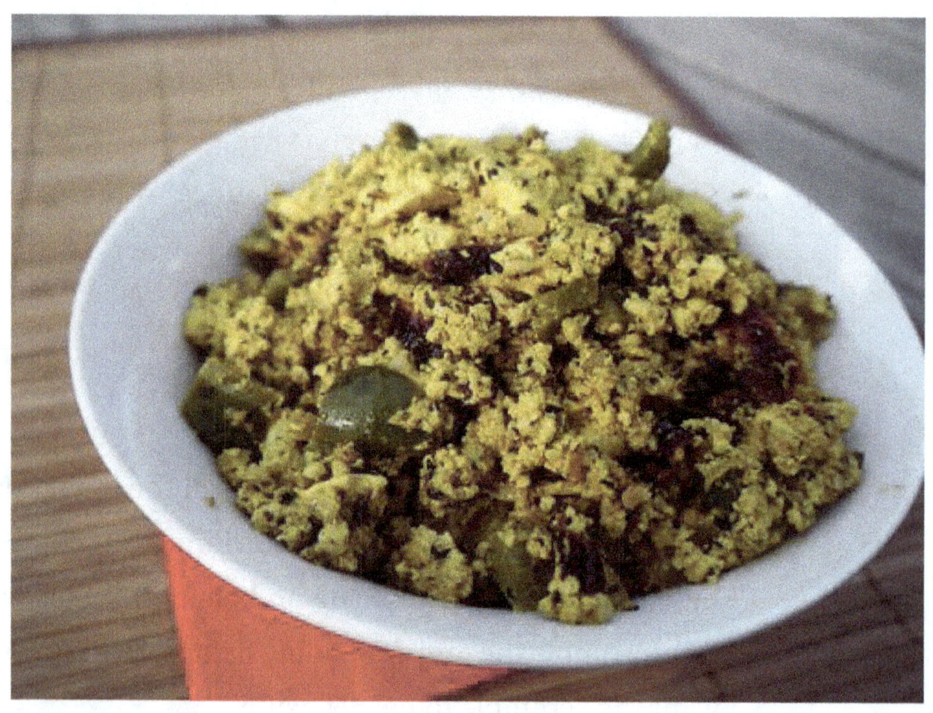

Quick Creamed Coconut Curry Spinach

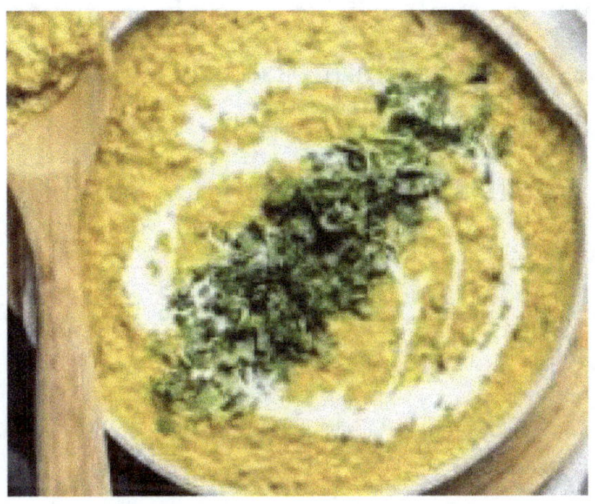

Preparation Time: 30 to 35minutes - Cooking Time: 5 minutes - Servings: 6

Ingredients:

- 1 small can whole fat coconut milk
- Cashews for garnish
- 2 ½ teaspoons yellow curry paste
- 1 pound frozen spinach, thawed and drained of moisture
- 1 ½ teaspoon lemon zest

Directions:

1. First of all, please certify you've all the ingredients out there. Please heat a medium-sized available. Please heat a medium-sized pan to medium-high heat, then add the curry paste & cook appropriately for about 30 to 40 seconds.

2. Then add a small amount of the coconut milk & stir to combine and then cook until the paste is aromatic.

3. This step is essential. Add the spinach, and then season.

4. Now quickly add the rest of the ingredients, apart from the cashews, & allow the sauce to reduce slightly.

5. One thing remains to be done. Keep the sauce creamy, but reduce it to coat the spinach thoroughly.

6. Finally, serve with chopped cashews.

Nutrition: Calories: 191 / Protein: 4g / Fat: 18g / Carbs: 3g

Vintage Moist Almond Cake

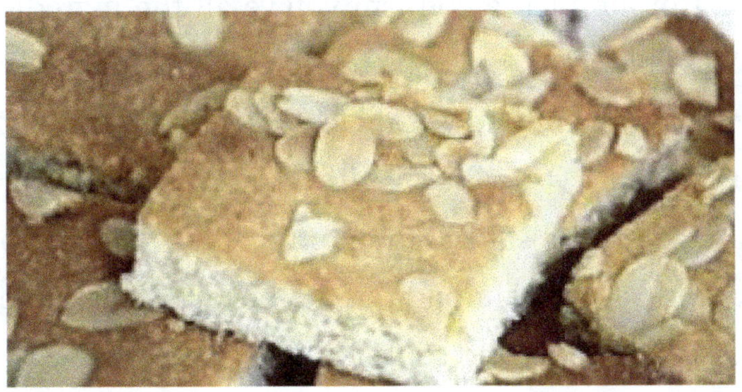

Preparation Time: 1 hour - Cooking Time: 30 minutes - Servings: 8

Ingredients:

- 5 oz. sugar
- 1 cup Greek yogurt, vanilla (full fat)
- 1 cup almond flour
- 1 ½ teaspoons baking powder
- 1 egg
- ¼ teaspoons baking soda
- 1 ½ teaspoons vanilla
- ¼ teaspoons salt
- 2 oz. butter (soft)
- ½ teaspoon cinnamon powder

Directions:

1. First of all, please confirm you've all the ingredients accessible. Grease a 0- inch layer cake tin and sprinkle with a little almond flour. Heat oven to about 3600 F. to 3700 F.

2. Now sift your salt, cinnamon powder, baking soda, baking powder, almond flour, & sugar in a large bowl. Stir to combine, and set aside.

3. This step is essential. Place in a blender, banana, egg, butter, sugar, and vanilla.

4. Then blend for about 2 minutes at super-speed; consistency should be smooth.

5. Pour blended mixture into almond flour mixture & mix thoroughly.

6. One thing remains to be done. Pour and scrape into the greased tin.

7. Finally, place in oven and bake for about 25 to 30 minutes. Cool & serve.

Nutrition: Calories: 157 / Protein: 2.3 g / Fat: 8 g / Carbs: 19.5 g

Iconic Braised Endives

Preparation Time: 20 to 25 minutes - Cooking Time: 35 minutes - Servings: 2

Ingredients:

- 1 ¾ oz. Butter
- Salt and pepper to taste
- 1 tablespoon Lemon juice
- 3 Endives(chopped lengthwise, brown bruised bits discarded)
- 3 ½ tablespoon Water

Directions:

1. First of all, please check that you've all the ingredients out there. Melt the butter in a non-stick place the endives in it.
2. Then season with salt and pepper & sprinkle the lemon juice on top.
3. One thing remains to be done. Now please leave to brown for about 5 to 10 minutes and then flip.
4. Finally, add a little water to the pan & cook covered for about 20 to 25 minutes.

Nutrition: Calories: 225 / Protein: 3 g / Fat: 21 g / Carbs: 9 g

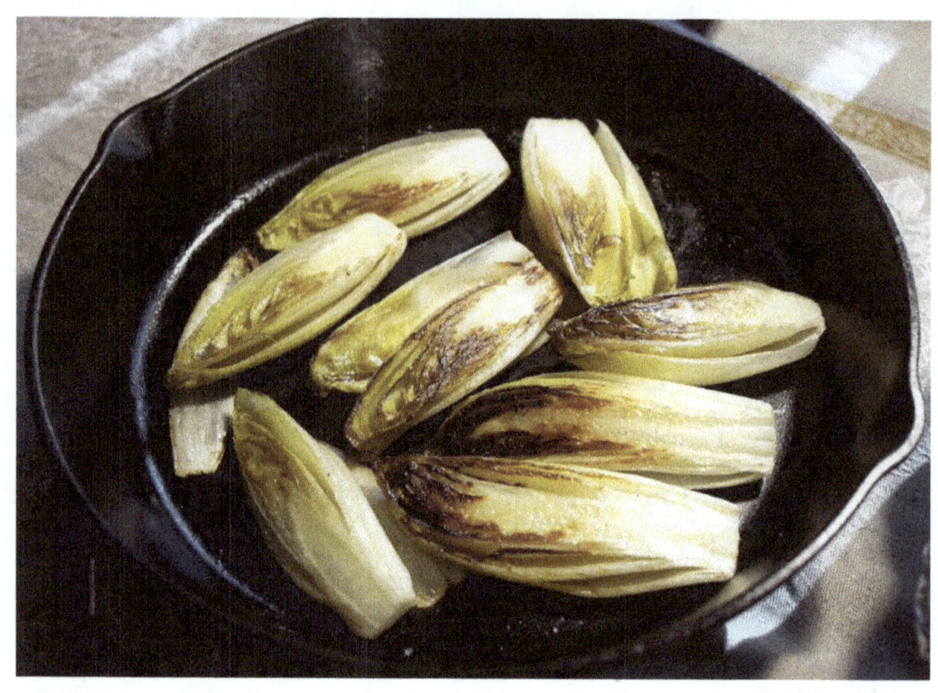